Purple Toolbox

Lose Weight Without a Plan or Diet

Written by
Ann Ashton Schilling

**FREE Coaching Session
with your Purchase
of this book – Thanks!**

Keep knocking, and the joy inside
will eventually open a window
and look out to see who's there. ~ Rumi

Cover design by Adrian Balint

Table of Contents

MIND

Where is Your Joy?

What Makes You Tick?

Who Do YOU Want to BE?

Smile!

You are NOT Alone!

Are You Living Your Truth?

Can You Raise Your Energy Frequency?

Do Thoughts Change Your Frequency?

Please Ask Questions

at

thepurpletoolbox@gmail.com

Thank you for reading

Purple Toolbox

Lose Weight Without a Plan or Diet

If you find this book to be helpful,

please take a moment to review it

at

Amazon.com

Thank you again!

Please look for the author's blog at

http://purpletoolbox.com

for additional Information and Tools

for

Thinner and Healthier Living

Please add Tags on Amazon.com

Introduction

Congratulations! If you are reading this, you have probably tried a variety of diet plans, weight loss schemes and over-the-counter supplements.

Many of your attempts were expensive, inconvenient and generally unhealthy. To make matters worse, none of your attempts was successful. The plans did not work...or, you were just not able to make them work for you. You felt like a failure.

Bottom line...your *bottom line... and your waistline...* did not change. The number on your scale did not change. You may have even gained a few pounds. You were disappointed in yourself. You asked, "What do I have to do to lose weight?"

The answer lies in understanding the real causes of weight gain which means understanding yourself.

The Purple Toolbox gives you the tools to understand your specific problem(s). It offers valuable advice to help you achieve healthy and sustainable weight loss.

Why Don't Diets Work?

Diets are torturous inventions of man (and woman) based on faulty science and greed. Much of the science they're based on is proven wrong eventually. Meanwhile, the many manufacturers make tons of money. And, most diets are ineffective.

Each claims to be the next big thing while repeating much of the same 'bull' you've heard before.

You have tried starving yourself and that lasted 3 days...and you gained a few pounds. You've tried one of those "extreme" work-out cd's ...one time. That was way too hard. You were hurting for a week.

When you combine starvation with exercise, your body actually goes into survival mode. Your metabolism slows down and it is almost impossible to lose weight. Your body perceives a catastrophe coming and it will hold on to your pounds to keep you alive.

You tried counting calories. What a pain that was writing down everything that you ate or drank. And, of course, you skipped a few things or lost your note book.

And, you ordered some of those packaged meals which tasted like their cardboard boxes. Yuk! The original nutrients were processed out of the so-called food. Then preservatives, dyes and other chemicals were added for indefinite shelf life.

Those make-believe foods are toxic because they do not provide the nutrition your body needs on a daily basis. They put a variety of poisons into your body, which your body has to work very hard to remove.

You have tried to eliminate fats from your diet. However, good fats are a very important part of your diet and are necessary for certain body functions...and for energy.

Last, but probably not least, you have tried to eliminate sugar from your diet by using artificial sweeteners and by drinking diet sodas. Again, no one is quite sure which is worse. Sugar and foods that turn quickly to sugar cause spikes in insulin levels. And, sugar is tremendously addictive. But, the chemicals in the sweeteners and sodas can have much worse side-effects.

The list goes on of all the fad diets that have come and gone over the years. They have gone because they were not effective. Let's dive into the problem further.

Why Are You Overweight?

For most of my coaching clients, food is a comfort. Food is a FIX for the distresses of life. They feel old, tired, unloved or they have physical ailments that cause pain somewhere in their bodies.

They say food helps to make them feel better. But, comfort foods, such as candy, cookies, ice cream...and even bread, are making them heavier. They feel worse. They eat more. It is a vicious cycle. Food (and, more specifically, sugar) has become an addiction.

Some just do not know what different types of foods do to or for your body. They have no knowledge of nutrition or chemistry. So, they make poor choices.

Some have developed diseases as a result of their poor diets. They rely on medications to try to control the symptoms. But, the side-effects from the medications make them feel even worse.

One common example is the over-use of sugar which has been shown to lead to diabetes. Diabetes requires using insulin to balance sugar levels in the body. That is another vicious cycle.

Those cycles have become almost epidemic in the United States. Over 60% of the adult population is very overweight or obese. The American Medical Association, for the first time, has declared OBESITY as a DISEASE. And, many children today are "off the charts" for their ages and on their way to being very overweight and very unhealthy.

One thing that most Americans do not know is that most of the wheat grown in the United States has been genetically altered to be more addictive. And, the wheat has virtually no nutritional value.

Most bread, pasta, cereals, cakes, cookies and other packaged foods taste good but they do not 'feed' your body. Most of those foods turn almost immediately to sugar, which causes insulin levels to rise.

As a result, your body's chemistry shifts in a dangerous way. If you are active, the sugar is somewhat reduced. If you are not, sugar causes inflammation which is the beginning of many diseases.

Excess sugar accumulates as fat. The most dangerous location is belly fat. Belly fat changes your hormonal levels and has been established as a precursor to a number of diseases, including diabetes and cancer.

The more you avoid those empty foods, the better your health.

There are so many other ways to "comfort" your body other than foods. We will explore some of those ways in the Toolbox. We will also explore the Good Foods that help your body instead of making it fat.

Do You Accumulate Stuff?

One of the common companions of fat accumulators is excess stuff. Not only do many of my clients accumulate pounds, they have other related addictions. They accumulate 'stuff'.

You hoard stuff that often you do not really need to make yourself feel better about the shortcomings that you have manufactured.

You may accumulate clothes, furniture, degrees, boyfriends, husbands or any number of things.

What are you accumulating? And, why are you accumulating stuff? What is it that you are missing or feel that you are missing?

In the Toolbox, we will search for answers to those questions.

Why Do You Do What You Do?

All of the "'holics" of this world are trying to make up for some unfortunate misperception that they are not "good enough" just the way they are. They are trying to fill some psychological gap...mostly from childhood experiences.

You abuse yourself with your obsession of choice. It may be alcohol, shopping, work, relationships, eating or many others.

When it comes to eating, a lot of people eat to hide their anguish, fear or anger. They hide behind the pounds.

Extra pounds 'protect' you from being hurt or abused by others...or, even by yourself.

Many of those misperceptions stem from your earliest memories. Well-intentioned parents, relatives or friends of the family may have uttered only a few words that have influenced your vision of who you are for your lifetime.

Many clients are amazed to learn that they are not unique in their childhood experiences. They are surprised that so many have obsessive tendencies.

We will explore ways to change your vision in the Toolbox Section of this book.

How Were You Programmed?

The way you are is a result of the way you were taught to think about yourself and the world around you. The way you are is also a result of your focus.

You were probably programmed by your parents, siblings and the people around you to think and feel a certain way...the way they did.

Or, you might have been the "black sheep" of the family because you did not go along with the program. You decided for yourself what you would do and how you would think about things. Somehow the guilt from that decision has followed you throughout your life.

You may have been taught to focus on negative, fear-based things. An example is a message like "Don't go out without your umbrella. You could catch your death." Every time you hear rain or see an umbrella, you shiver.

A more positive approach would result in your thinking, "The rain will bring flowers and fill the streams and lakes."

Positive thinking will empower you, inspire you.

What would you do if you knew you could change? Most clients never realized there was a choice. They have stayed stuck all of their lives. They thought that was just the way they were and they could not change it.

The Good News is that you can change your programming. You can change the way you think. You can change your focus. There are tools in the Purple Toolbox for that, too!

Simple Weight Loss Concept

The simple concept of this book and the Purple Toolbox is that all aspects of you (Mind, Body and Spirit) have to be in balance for any new adventure to succeed.

When you address the issues that have kept you unhappy, you will be able to more easily reach your goals, including losing weight.

This book will help you to understand who you are, how you fit into your own vision and how you think you should look. Your vision of yourself can change. Your body image can change.

You can change. The Purple Toolbox is full of ideas and concepts that will support you in changing any aspect of your life, including losing weight.

What If?

This book and the Purple Toolbox provide tools to make the life you are living better in many ways...no matter what your present circumstances.

Now is the time to prepare for a more loving, creative, energetic life. You can live a life of Vision, Expression and Success. Being a slimmer you will happen naturally when you are in balance. Make a few small changes and see how you look and feel.

BE open to learning or re-learning some techniques that you can use to be happier right now and in the future...wherever that future takes you...or where you take it.

Wherever you focus, energy follows. What if you took just one small step...and then another. Read on for the tools to help you.

Purple Toolbox

The Purple Toolbox is divided into three sections to serve the different aspects of you – Mind, Body and Spirit.

First, your MIND must be focused on what you desire in your life. You can spend years wasting time rehashing all the mistakes and "What-Ifs" of your life. Or, you can focus on what you want to create next.

At any moment in time you can create a new BODY. You cannot do much about your height. However, just about every other aspect of your body can be changed. The Purple Toolbox has tools to help you.

Your SPIRIT patiently awaits your attention. If you are like most people, you get caught up in the day-to-day aspects of living and only occasionally acknowledge your spiritual side. In just a few minutes a day you can change your life. Read on...

MIND

Where is Your Joy?

I quoted the 13th century poet Rumi at the beginning of this book.

Keep knocking, and the joy inside
will eventually open a window
and look out to see who's there. ~ Rumi

Have you found the joy in you?

Most of us spend so much of our lives taking care of the little time-consuming details that we do not find the joy within ourselves. If you have not found the joy in you, you will do other things to make yourself feel good...like eat...and other addictive behaviors.

Find the thing (or maybe a few things) that makes you unique. You were born with gifts. What are they?

Do some soul searching. List the things that made you feel special?

Are you funny? Can you tell a joke?
Do you care more than most?
Do you love yourself?
Do you love animals? Nature?
Do you love the planet?
Do you like to write? Paint?
Do you like helping people?
Do you love the challenge of creating businesses?

Find the thing that makes you special and create from that space.

That is where you will find the JOY in your life.

You say, "It's too late. I'm too old!"

It is never too late to share your gifts with yourself and with the world. That is where you will nurture yourself and others. You BEing YOU is where you will find your JOY!

What Makes You Tick?

What is your earliest self-image based on the set of values that you learned at home? For example, did you feel like a leader or a follower? Were you outgoing or shy? Did you laugh or cry? Were you happy or angry?

An important tool is RE-EVALUATION.

You have internalized the values and opinions of others formed during childhood. Now is the time for a reexamination.

Examine your priorities. The value or need that motivates you and where you place your focus determines the direction of your life.

What makes you happy? What do you do for fun? What gives meaning to your life? What is your purpose? Where do you find your joy?

What makes you want to sit on your couch and eat ice cream? Do you think of Ben and Jerry as relatives?

These questions are tools to help you start the conversation with yourself.

Some examples of values:

Dependence – Feelings you have for parents, family

Independence – Spreading your wings, trying new ideas

Self-worth – Pride in yourself, your gifts and accomplishments

Love – Feeling connected to yourself and others

Spend some time thinking about which of those needs is most important to YOU. It will give you some insight into why you do what you do.

The good news is that you can change your life by changing your focus.

Who Do YOU Want to Be?

Are you happy in your own skin? Are you content?

Or, are you confused and disappointed with your life of pain and struggle? Does your reality match the vision that you have for your life? Do YOU look like your VISION of you?

If you are, in fact, a child of God (or Creator) why isn't your life one of pure joy? Why do tragedies happen? Why do you lose loved ones? Why are you sick and miserable? Why are you fat?

Do you want to remember your Spiritual Nature? Do you want to BE Love, Peace and Joy?

Why can you not BE what you choose to BE?

You just have to believe that you are that.

Try meditating.

Sit quietly, breathing slowly. Visualize your breath. As you become quiet, try to connect with your soul. Ask your soul how it is doing. Then, just listen.

Ask what you can do to connect with your soul and to help it. Then, just listen. Listen for answers, expecting that they will come. Then...

PICTURE YOU PERFECT! You are that!

Try this for as little as a few minutes each day. Afterwards, write down any ideas or messages that 'pop' into your head. Expand this practice as needed.

As you believe on the inside, you will project that joyous creation on the outside. You will glow with Love and radiant energy.

SMILE!

Smiling has an amazing effect on how you feel.

When you smile, you lift hundreds of tiny muscles in your face and head. It is an instant face lift.

And, smiling fools the brain into thinking that you are happy...even if you are not.

Smiling for even a minute can lift your spirits. If you remember to smile throughout the day, you will notice people smiling back at you. Smiling is contagious.

You will love how you feel. And, you will make other people around you feel good, too.

Try this experiment for just one day. Set your watch, clock or cell phone to ring every hour. Every hour smile for just one minute. At the end of the day, look back and think about how that felt.

My guess is that you have just begun a new, very beneficial habit.

You are NOT Alone!

You were born alone and you will die alone. That is a fact. However, we are all together in that experience.

Think back through all the many people you have met in your life. Every person changed you just a little bit or a lot.

Every day and every encounter was a new chapter. People stayed for a moment or for years. People taught you lessons. Or, you taught them.

Take some time to review some of your most important relationships. What were the lessons you learned? What do you think were the lessons you taught the other person?

Try to see yourself through that person's eyes? What do you think he or she saw? How did you change? How did he or she change?

Look for the lessons. Look for the trends.

You may have repeatedly dated the same person over and over again – in a different body – because you did not GET the lesson.

For women, it is usually a father figure that did not meet your expectations. He did not give you the love you desired or deserved.

For men, it is usually a mother figure who did not meet expectations.

Most of us have spent too much time looking outside ourselves for what we think we are missing. But, it has been there all along. Love is within you.

You have one life. Love it! Laugh through it! Live it! Be the treasure you are seeking.

Are You Living Your Truth?

Truth generally means "being in accordance with reality."

However, reality varies from person to person. Your reality, your knowledge of the facts regarding just about anything, can be quite different from mine. Your reality can be very different from just about anyone else's truth.

When you rely on someone else's truth to guide you, you are living a lie. You are giving away your power.

Without getting too philosophic, the one person you can rely on is yourself.

As the energy of every new day presents itself, you may feel different. You may find yourself with a very new perspective. Your truth may shift in a very big way.

Search within yourself whenever you feel the urge. As you search within, you will be inspired in new ways to create a new reality for yourself. Take back your power from all those who have taken it from you.

The new reality you create for yourself will be Your Truth! Acknowledge it. Live it. Be it.

BODY

How Can You Improve Your Health Easily?

Health is that state when all (or most of) the systems of your body are working in harmony. That state is called homeostasis.

More technically put, (according to the American Heritage Dictionary) homeostasis is a state of physiological equilibrium produced by a balance of functions and chemical composition within an organism.

Many factors contribute to ultimate health. Probably the primary factor is the way you think about your health.

If you think that everyone gets sick as they age, that is what you will experience in your life. It is a self-fulfilling prophecy.

If you think that your health will remain perfect and that any little ailments can be healed naturally, that is what you will experience. Again, it is a self-fulfilling prophecy.

By changing the way you think, you take a huge step toward changing your current health situation.

Your energy renews itself continuously, both mentally and physically. You can use that continuous flow of energy to modify health issues as well many other issues in your life.

Some people feel that if you have an ailment, a "medication" will make you better. However, there are many ways that you can improve your health without medications.

First, recognize that every pill has a little poison in it. There have been many books written about the overuse of medications and how they, in fact, actually keep your body from healing itself.

There are many natural remedies that you can use to treat conditions. Some mentioned in this book include Homeopathy, Essential Oils, Raising Your Frequency, Visualization and Crystals.

And, what you put in your mouth in the way of food and drink makes a huge impact on your health. Simply put, the more one ingredient foods you eat, the better your health will be.

One ingredient foods are simple, unprocessed foods that are in their natural state (or as close to it as possible). Examples are organic chicken and grass-fed beef, wild fish, fresh vegetables, fresh fruits, sweet potatoes, fresh herbs, nuts, seeds and oils (virgin olive, avocado and coconut oils). And, of course, water that is free of chemicals is also a necessity.

Foods that will cause you to age prematurely and will also cause disease include wheat (even whole wheat) and gluten, high fructose corn syrup, sugar and foods like white potatoes that change to sugar, soybean oil and other highly processed vegetable oils...and basically anything in a box or a can.

Dr. Joel Fuhrman suggests that if you eat one fresh mushroom and some onion each day you will cut your chances of having heart issues and cancer by over 80%. I like those odds.

Visit www.purpletoolbox.com for information on herbs and amino acids that will help you.

Avoid eating microwaved foods. Those ovens are banned in Russia and many other parts of the world. Instead sauté anything quickly in an enamel pan.

Simple changes can produce amazing results.

Stop Reading Labels!

Eat foods that don't have any. The more fresh foods you eat that have no labels the better. The more organic, locally grown or personally grown foods without pesticides and hormones you eat the better.

Probably the best news about eating fresh foods is that you can eat almost limitless amounts. You will not be hungry and your body will be getting the nutrition it needs. There is no diet here. There is only a lifestyle change...a very tasty lifestyle change.

Of course, there are certain foods that are more beneficial than others. I will list below my favorites.

When you are looking for food, remember the saying, ""YOU are what you EAT." Find nutritious foods at a local farmers' market, in your own backyard (or balcony) or at a food store.

If you are limited to your local food store, shop the perimeter of the store. That is where you will find fresh items as opposed to processed non-foods (in the middle aisles).

Vegetables

Organic or farm-grown Spinach
Organic Spring Mixed Salad
Romaine Lettuce
Kale
Broccoli
Green Beans
Sugar Snap Peas
Carrots
Mini Carrots (great snack)
Tomatoes
Cucumbers
Zucchini
Green, Red and Yellow Peppers
Hot Peppers
Beets
Corn
Sweet Potatoes
Yams
Pumpkins
Mushrooms
Onions
Garlic

Fruits

Blueberries
Strawberries
Raspberries
Cherries
Grapes
Kiwi
Apples
Oranges
Mangos
Bananas (one per day)
Cantalope
Honeydew Melon
Lemons (disinfects your home, too)
Limes

Organic or Natural Dairy

Organic Milk
Organic Cage-Free or Omega 3 Eggs
Organic Butter
Organic or Natural Cheeses
Organic Greek Yogurt

All Natural or Organic Meats

Organic Chicken

Grass Fed Beef

Fresh or Frozen Fish

Non-farm raised Salmon

Miscellaneous

Dark Chocolate

Olive Oil – Black Bottle with Press Date

Steel Cut Oatmeal

Organic or Natural Maple Syrup
Stevia Natural Sweetener

Red Wine – French Rabbit Pino Noir in a box

Organic Sliced Almonds
Organic Walnuts

Herbs - Grow these on your windowsill
       Basil
       Mint
       Sage
       Basil
       Rosemary
       Thyme

Water – Filtration System or Buy Gallons of Spring Water and refill smaller bottles as needed.

There are no "Cheat Days." No calorie counting. Every one of the food mentioned here feeds the body in certain, unique ways.

Many of my clients have lost ten pounds or more in a week just eliminating wheat from their diets and substituting lots of vegetables and fruits. They were not hungry!

Try different foods. Mix it up. Enjoy!

Muscle or Fat?

Muscle makes you look better than fat. It burns more calories than fat. Muscle also supports your bone structure by keeping your bones and joints in place. And, muscle BUILDS YOUR BONES.

When you lift any kind of weight, even soup cans, the muscle puts tension on the bone which causes the bone to grow. The more tension that you put on your muscles, the more your bones will increase in strength.

If you spend only a few minutes (5 to 15) every other day lifting light weights, you will feel stronger and healthier.

My friend Charles Garcia, who is a professional trainer, states often, "Your mind tells you where you want to go. Your bones and muscles get you there, if they are able."

On your off days, MOVE for 5 to 15 minutes. Walk, dance, swim or do some other form of

exercise. If you have more time, use an elliptical machine or do yoga, ti chi, palates or Shun Tao.

Just move!

Even if you are confined to a wheelchair, move some part of your body. Move your toes, your feet, and your arms. Contract your muscles.

As you move, your lungs will breathe in more oxygen. The fluids in your body that nourish your cells will move. Your blood and your lymph will transport nutrition to more of your body. Your energy levels will increase. Your mind will work better.

You will feel better with just that small amount of exercise. Try it for a week. Increase the time as needed.

And, of course, check with your doctor before beginning any kind of exercise.

Can You Raise Your Energetic Frequency?

Frequency is the measurable rate of steady electrical energy flow between two points. Everything has frequency. Every cell in your body has a frequency.

One of the simplest ways that anyone can raise his or her energetic frequency is with ESSENTIAL OILS.

Therapeutic Grade Essential Oils have the highest frequency of any natural substance known to man according to clinical research.

And, because of their amazingly high frequencies, essential oils create an environment where *disease cannot live*.

Essential oils also align frequencies to balance and harmonize body organs. Additionally, high frequencies also boost activity in the brain and other organs and would therefore support capabilities on many levels.

All atoms in the universe have motion. Each episodic motion has a "frequency" (the number of oscillations per second) which is measured in Hertz:

1 Hertz (Hz) = 1 oscillation per second (ops)
1 Kilo Hertz (KHz) = 1,000 ops
1 Mega Hertz (MHz) = 1,000,000 ops

The average Human Body has a range of 62-78 MHz (Mega Hertz). If your body's frequency goes below about 58 MHz, you will be susceptible to disease. You will be receptive to CANCER at 42MHz. You are vulnerable to DEATH at 25MHz.

So, how do you feed your body? Most people in this age of fast food feed their bodies with processed or canned foods, which have 0 Hz. Processed foods, then, are not really feeding your body. They are filling you stomach and, if anything, draining energy from your body as the food is digested.

Fresh Foods and Herbs have frequencies that

range from 20 - 27 Hz. Dried Foods and Herbs range from 15 - 22 Hz.
Essential oils' frequencies start at 52 Hz and go as high as 320 Hz, the frequency of rose oil. Lavender oil has a frequency of 118 Hz. I would suggest that Essential Oils should be an essential part of everyone's health regimen.

Visit http://www.heavenscentoils.net/ for more information.

Do Thoughts Change Your Frequency?

Absolutely!

It has been found during studies of frequency that the thoughts going through a participant's mind created a noticeable difference in frequency.

The more positive the thoughts, the higher the frequency readings become. Those whose thoughts focused on Prayer or Meditation had the highest frequencies.

In other words, if the participants were able to 'get out of their minds' and pray or meditate with their hearts, their results were substantially higher.

Positive thoughts during testing raised the frequency in the body significantly.

Negative thoughts during testing lowered the body frequency considerably.

Meditation and Prayer increased frequencies more than just positive thoughts.

Can You Talk to Your Body?

How about not only talking to your body, parts of your body and organs? How about talking to your cells?

Every cell in your body has energy and what some would call a 'soul.' Why could you not talk to your cells? And, why would they not respond?

Talk to your skin. Talk to your organs. You can even think the thoughts...you do not actually have to say the words. Say in your mind what result you would like.

If you have imperfections or some signs of age that you would rather have gone away...just tell them to go away.

Try it. It works!

Will Homeopathy Improve Your Health?

Homeopathy is a type of medical treatment that uses minute doses of remedies that in massive doses would cause the symptoms similar to the disease being treated.

Homeopathy is used around the world to effectively treat an amazingly wide variety of ailments without the side effects of many medications.

Most health food stores can help you to determine a good homeopathic treatment for what ails you. And, there are books and resources in health food stores, book stores and online.

SPIRIT

Can You Love Yourself?

Love is your birthright. It is that warm, fuzzy feeling that you experienced when you were held for the very first time.

On the day of your birth, the cold and light of day was a shock. But, then warm arms and a warm body held you close. You felt a heartbeat. Wow! It sounded just like the one you heard for the nine months you were growing in your mother's belly before you were born.

Growing up, perhaps your parents weren't the most loving people. But, there was always a caring grandmother or teacher to hold your hand and who would encourage you to "Do your best" or "Be your best." As your interests expanded, there were others who encouraged you along your journey.

As you grew older, you found friends and supporters who mirrored the love within you. They would encourage you to push yourself in a positive direction.

You can do that for you. And, now is the time to do it.

According to numerology, 2013 is a 33/6 year with spiritual gifts. That means that the year 2013 is a very positive year about vision and expression. If you flow with the energy, you will see the value in yourself and sense it in others. Spiritual energy will be available for you to help you serve yourself and serve others.

The year 2014 is a 34/7 year with spiritual gifts. During 2014, trust in the spiritual process, stability and the expressiveness flowing around you. It is a great year for self-discovery.

When you quiet yourself, you will sense the love within you. Your soul is pure love. And, you will connect with your soul (or spirit) through prayer, thought or meditation.

The experience will be similar to times in the past when you felt the love within you. However, you will feel yourself changing. You will be able to create new experiences in your life.

You will be able to let go of negative situations that do not support you. You will create new experiences that are much more positive. You will be the creator of your outcomes. You will not be the victim anymore.

You will do that by connecting on a higher level with your soul enabled by new levels of energy.

The more you strengthen that connection with your soul – that true love connection – the more joy you will feel. You will radiate love.

And, what you radiate or project is what you will attract into your life. When you radiate love, you attract love. You will be surrounded by loving people.

Try it! You will adore how you feel.
You will magically attract people, events and circumstances that will create even more love and joy in your life.

One way to keep track of your progress is to carry a small journal or notebook with you. Jot down your reactions to situations. Note how you feel about how you 'handle' events or people. Think briefly about how you might improve and how you might serve others in a more loving way. How might you better serve yourself?

A journal helps you see where you might be more positive and loving. It also shows you how impressive you are. Where do you 'WOW' yourself?

Can You Create a New Consciousness?

Of course! Through meditation, you can get in touch with the spiritual side of you. The true nature of you does not worry or get angry. Your true nature just IS. If you learn to get past all the mundane 'stuff' that keeps your mind occupied most of the time, you will find a magnificent you.

You will thrive in the new environment that you create. You will welcome new levels of consciousness that allow for higher achievements in all areas of your life.

You will reach a New Energy.

Your new energy, full of love and wisdom, will support you to be beautiful in all ways. Your mind, spirit and body will carry you to BE the perfect you.

Read on to see how this new concept works to create the perfect you.

Do Breath Control and Meditation Heal?

A strange question you say?

What if there were spaces between your breaths where you could rest and just BE you? No anger, no emotions...just you?

Try breathing in slowly and deeply. Then, breathe out slowly, relaxing.

As you reach that place where you have breathed out totally and you have not yet breathed in again, relax totally and feel the peace that is YOU.

Stay in that space as long as you can, feeling the peace and the nothingness.

Repeat several times.

This little exercise can be a very nice beginning to a meditation...or, it can calm you in the middle of a difficult day at work.

It can take you from negative energy to neutral...and then to positive. So, it will raise your frequency or vibration.

The REAL YOU has a higher frequency than the angry, stressed out you. And, the more you practice this type of breathing the more you will reconnect with the REAL YOU!

What Results Can ASKING Achieve?

Whether you call it praying or meditating (or, some other form of dialogue), you are communicating with someone or something outside yourself whom you probably feel is listening to you.

Have you ASKED for what you need and want?

Have you asked really *knowing* that your request would be answered?

And, then have you *blessed your request* and let it go?

That is the way to ASK! There are many 'beings' out there listening for our requests. And, the GOOD NEWS is that they will always answer. They must! It is a cosmic law.

However, the answer might not be exactly

what you expected. Be open to the results.

Those beings include (but are not limited to) God (or Creator), Mother Mary, Jesus (or Jeshua), angels, guides, spirit guides, ascended masters, the elohim, archangels and elementals. Just know that they are listening and that they also offer help in a myriad of ways.

If you have a problem or would like help with something (like driving your car, writing a complicated paper or RAISING YOUR FREQUENCY) just ask.

Then, rest knowing that help is on the way!

Life is Like a River?

If you think of life as a river, how do you view that river? How do you react to it? How do you feel about it?

You can stand on the bank of the river and watch it flow by. You wonder how the water would feel on your legs. What other creatures and things are in the water?

You can wade into the river and feel the river flow around you and past you. You can watch as leaves and twigs flow by. You can imagine the other lifeforms under the surface.

You can float along with the flow of the river and see where it takes you. You can feel the current moving you and watch it push other things alongside you.

Or, you can decide where and how you want to go and use your mind and body to take you

there. You may want to go across the
river...or, against the current.

Use your mind to set a goal. Use your spirit
and creativity to make plans. Then, use your
body to get you there.

You are so capable of so many things. Use the
resources you were given to guide you and
take you where you want to go.

Probably, the most difficult part of that
scenario is deciding what it is that you desire
or where you want to go.

If you could wave a "magic" wand, who would
you be and where would you be? What would
you dream for you?

You have a magic wand. Use your mind and
your spirit working together to decide where
and who you want to be. Let them do their
magic. Dream!

What If You Could Heal Yourself?

Jesus said, "According to your faith be it done to you." (Matthew 9:29)

Do you believe you are a child of God (or a Higher Power)? Do you believe that it is your legacy to be able to heal yourself? Or, do you rely on doctors and medications to heal you?

I know that is a stretch for some people. The dark have tried to control you to the extent that you would not remember who you are and what talents you possess.

Now is the time to start remembering who you are. You are an expression of God - of His consciousness – and of your soul. You can connect with Him and your soul whenever you would like just by willing to or intending to make that connection.

You - as a part of God - can create and you can

heal. You can manifest whatever you desire - according to your belief.

Jesus told you so!

What are the Benefits of Visualization?

There are many books and courses that focus on visualization. Simply put, you enter a state of relaxation or meditation and 'see yourself' Being, Doing or Having something you would like to BE, do or have.

One way to be more creative in the process is visualizing the INFINITY sign, which is a sideways figure eight. Imagine the number '8' on its side. Now imagine that each loop of the infinity sign represents either the male or the female aspect of you.

As you 'see' a line flowing around the shape, you are integrating the two aspects of you that are at times at odds with each other.

When you integrate the male and the female of you, you become more creative and more powerful. Try it! And, then visualize what you would like to BE, do or have. Visualize you at a HIGHER FREQUENCY!

Can Crystals Help Your Health?

Crystals have wonderful properties that can raise your body's frequency and, according to the type of crystal or healing gem, offer you help in many ways.

To give you an idea of how they work, here is a short list of crystals and healing stones with simple descriptions of their properties.

Amethyst	- Healing, Psychic Ability
Angelite	- Higher self, Telepathy
Citrine	- Manifestation, Power
Jade	- Health, Wealth, Love
Jasper	- Self-love, Protection
Lapis	Total Awareness
Moonstone	- Intuition
Rose Quartz	- Attract Love
Topaz	- Life Purpose, Metabolism

To choose a stone, hold it. Then, ask the stone if it can help you with a certain desire.

Generally, if you begin to fall forward, the answer is "Yes." And, if you begin to fall backward, the answer is "No." You can test how your body reacts by trying a few stones.

Keep trying different crystals or stones until you feel a very positive response.

For more information about crystals and gemstones, visit http://www.blackmountainbead.com .

What's Next?

Your CHOICE!

Which of the ideas presented here resonates with you?

Which Tools motivate you to DO something? What will you do? Choose one idea or one technique. Try that one idea for a few days. See how you feel. Sense how your thinking has changed...or not. Notice new results in your life.

Try something else or add another technique to your routine. Set aside just a few minutes a day for you to explore you and some new ideas.

Many of my clients find that working alone with the Toolbox is very difficult.

As her gift to you for purchasing this book, Ann is offering a *FREE Coaching Session.*

Please contact Ann at *thepurpletoolbox@gmail.com* *for an appointment.*

She looks forward to hearing from you.

About the Author

Ann Ashton Schilling is a published author, healer, coach and media consultant. She has helped many hundreds of clients to remove physical and emotional pain so they can lose weight and focus on their power and creativity.

She has pursued mastery in many modalities, including Reiki, Matrix Energetics, Quantum-Touch and many other natural approaches to health. She has amazed audiences by removing pain from participants right on stage.

Ann looks for ways to help others find their own path to health. Your body is your vision of yourself. She presents tools that will help you 'see'the Magnificent You.

If she can be of help to you, contact her at~

thepurpletoolbox@gmail.com

She welcomes comments and questions. Your question may result in a future book.

As her gift to you for purchasing this book, she offers a **FREE Coaching Session** to help you to Celebrate YOU!

www.ingramcontent.com/pod-product-compliance
Lightning Source LLC
Chambersburg PA
CBHW070603290526
45790CB00002B/763